HEAL YOUR KIDNEYS

A HOLISTIC APPROACH TO DETOX, REPAIR, AND OPTIMAL KIDNEY HEALTH

TABLE OF CONTENTS

CHAPTER ONE

INTRODUCTION TO KIDNEY HEALTH

1.1 THE ROLE OF KIDNEYS IN THE BODY

The kidneys are two vital, bean-shaped organs that are situated on either side of your spine, just below the ribcage. Despite their small size—each kidney being about the size of a fist—they perform an incredibly important function within the body. These organs play a crucial role in maintaining the body's internal environment, ensuring homeostasis (balance) across various physiological processes.

At the core of kidney function is the filtration of blood. Each kidney contains approximately one million tiny filtering units called nephrons. These nephrons filter out waste products, toxins, excess water, and electrolytes, which are then excreted as urine. The kidneys are responsible for eliminating metabolic byproducts like urea and creatinine, which result from normal cellular processes in the body. By maintaining a healthy balance of electrolytes such as sodium, potassium, and calcium, the kidneys help regulate blood pressure and prevent imbalances that could otherwise disrupt the functioning of cells, tissues, and organs.

In addition to filtration, kidneys also play a role in regulating fluid balance. They control how much water is retained or expelled from the body, which is vital for proper hydration. The kidneys' ability to adjust the amount of water excreted based on the body's needs ensures that the bloodstream maintains the optimal viscosity for nutrient transport and waste removal.

Beyond filtration, the kidneys have an endocrine function—they produce and release important hormones that help regulate other bodily processes. For instance, the kidneys secrete erythropoietin, which stimulates the production of red blood cells in the bone marrow in response to low oxygen levels. Additionally, they produce renin, which helps regulate blood pressure, and active vitamin D, which plays a role in calcium and phosphate metabolism.

1.2 UNDERSTANDING KIDNEY FUNCTION AND COMMON ISSUES

Kidney function is often assessed by examining several key indicators, such as the glomerular filtration rate (GFR), urine output, and blood levels of waste products like creatinine. A decline in kidney function is a gradual process, often undetected until a significant amount of kidney damage has occurred. The kidneys are remarkably resilient, and even when one kidney is damaged, the other can compensate for its loss. However, when both kidneys begin to fail, the consequences can be severe, leading to life-threatening conditions.

Some of the most common kidney issues include:

- **Chronic Kidney Disease (CKD):** CKD is a progressive condition in which kidney function deteriorates over time, often as a result of diabetes, hypertension, or certain genetic conditions. This condition is typically silent in its early stages, with few noticeable symptoms, which makes it particularly dangerous. By the time people experience symptoms such as fatigue, swelling, and changes in urine output, significant kidney damage may have already occurred.

- **Acute Kidney Injury (AKI):** Unlike CKD, AKI is a sudden and often reversible condition in which the kidneys lose their ability to filter waste. This can be caused by a variety of factors, including dehydration, infections, medications, or physical trauma. While AKI is more urgent and acute, with appropriate treatment, kidney function can often be restored.

- **Kidney Stones:** Kidney stones are hard deposits of minerals and salts that form in the kidneys and can block the urinary tract, causing intense pain, urinary issues, and sometimes kidney damage if not treated promptly. They often form due to dehydration, high salt intake, or metabolic imbalances.

- **Polycystic Kidney Disease (PKD):** PKD is a genetic disorder in which fluid-filled cysts grow in the kidneys, eventually leading to kidney enlargement and compromised function. Over time, PKD can lead to CKD.

- **Urinary Tract Infections (UTIs):** UTIs can affect the kidneys if they spread to the renal system. Infections like pyelonephritis can cause pain, fever, and kidney damage if not treated effectively.

While these issues represent some of the most common kidney problems, the kidney's ability to function under stress and repair itself is remarkable. However, the kidneys' capacity for repair diminishes as the damage becomes more severe, making early detection and prevention crucial for preserving long-term kidney health.

1.3 WHY KIDNEY HEALTH MATTERS FOR OVERALL WELL-BEING

The importance of kidney health cannot be overstated. Kidneys are involved in so many critical functions that their decline can affect virtually every system in the body. When kidney function diminishes, toxins and waste products accumulate in the bloodstream, causing a variety of symptoms ranging from fatigue and weakness to confusion and nausea. The accumulation of these toxins can lead to a state of toxicity, which negatively impacts the immune system, digestive system, and even the brain.

Proper kidney function is essential for maintaining blood pressure. The kidneys help regulate blood pressure by controlling the volume of fluid and the balance of sodium in the blood. When the kidneys are damaged, they are less able to filter excess salt, leading to fluid retention, increased blood pressure, and the risk of cardiovascular diseases. High blood pressure is, in fact, both a cause and a consequence of kidney disease. It's a vicious cycle where high blood pressure can damage the kidneys, and kidney disease can, in turn, worsen high blood pressure.

Kidneys also have an essential role in bone health. They regulate the levels of calcium and phosphate in the body and activate vitamin D, which is necessary for calcium absorption in the gut. A malfunctioning kidney may lead to an imbalance of these minerals, increasing the risk of bone diseases such as osteoporosis and fractures.

Furthermore, healthy kidneys produce erythropoietin, which stimulates the bone marrow to produce red blood cells. When kidney function declines, this hormone is produced in insufficient amounts, leading to anemia. Anemia, in turn, contributes to fatigue, weakness, and poor circulation, significantly diminishing a person's quality of life.

The importance of maintaining kidney health is also related to managing other chronic conditions. For individuals with diabetes, hypertension, or cardiovascular diseases, protecting kidney function is a key part of managing overall health. Chronic kidney disease (CKD) can accelerate the progression of other diseases, leading to complications and additional health problems. Maintaining kidney health is crucial for preventing the long-term effects of these conditions.

Finally, kidney health directly impacts the body's ability to detoxify. As the primary organ responsible for filtering waste and excess substances, the kidneys contribute significantly to the body's natural detoxification process. A compromised kidney system can lead to the accumulation of toxins, which may cause inflammation, stress on organs, and a weakened immune system. Detoxifying through proper kidney care is not only important for those with existing kidney issues but also for preventing long-term damage to the body.

CHAPTER TWO

THE SCIENCE BEHIND KIDNEY DETOXIFICATION

2.1 HOW KIDNEYS FILTER AND DETOXIFY

The kidneys are the body's natural filtration and detoxification system, working tirelessly to remove waste products, excess substances, and toxins from the bloodstream. Each kidney contains about a million functional units called nephrons, which are responsible for the filtration process. The nephron is composed of several key parts, including the glomerulus (a network of tiny capillaries) and the tubules (which carry filtered substances). These components work together to ensure that blood is filtered efficiently.

Blood enters the kidneys through the renal artery, which divides into smaller blood vessels, ultimately reaching the glomerulus. The glomerulus functions as a filter, allowing small molecules, waste products, and excess water to pass into the nephron's tubules while preventing larger molecules like proteins and blood cells from being lost. The filtered liquid, called the filtrate, contains waste products, electrolytes, and water.

Once the filtrate enters the tubules, it undergoes further processing. The tubules have the ability to reabsorb substances that the body needs to keep, such as glucose, amino acids, and most electrolytes. This reabsorption process helps the kidneys maintain the balance of essential nutrients in the blood. What remains in the tubules after this reabsorption process is the final urine, which contains waste, toxins, excess water, and other substances the body needs to eliminate. The urine then travels through the renal pelvis, down the ureters, and into the bladder, where it is stored until it is ready to be excreted.

In addition to filtering waste, the kidneys also play a role in detoxifying harmful substances. The kidneys filter out drugs, environmental toxins, metabolic byproducts, and chemicals that enter the body through food, air, or skin. The process of detoxification is not only about waste removal but also involves the kidneys neutralizing or breaking down certain harmful compounds. This detoxification process involves a series of enzymatic reactions, particularly in the liver and kidneys, where substances are converted into water-soluble compounds that can be easily excreted through urine.

The kidneys also regulate the balance of electrolytes and acid-base levels, which are essential for maintaining overall body health. They help neutralize acids in the bloodstream by secreting hydrogen ions into the urine and reabsorbing bicarbonate to maintain a healthy pH level in the body. By performing these tasks, kidneys are critical to keeping the body's internal environment stable and functioning optimally.

2.2 THE IMPORTANCE OF DETOXING FOR KIDNEY HEALTH

Kidneys are designed to detoxify and filter out waste, but like any other system in the body, they can become overburdened with time. The process of detoxifying the kidneys is important because it helps prevent the accumulation of harmful substances that can damage these vital organs. When the kidneys are overloaded with toxins, they may not function properly, leading to a condition known as kidney dysfunction or disease.

Detoxing is essential for kidney health because it aids in preventing damage caused by waste buildup, reduces the risk of developing kidney stones, and can even help to reverse early stages of kidney disease. The kidneys naturally detoxify the body on a daily basis, but due to factors like a poor diet, exposure to toxins, stress, lack of hydration, and certain medications, the kidneys can become sluggish or overwhelmed, leading to impaired detoxification.

Detoxing the kidneys helps them operate at peak efficiency by supporting their natural filtration and detoxification abilities. A clean, well-functioning kidney system means that the body can efficiently remove toxins, reducing the burden on other organs such as the liver, which also plays a critical role in detoxification. Detoxification supports the kidneys in performing their key functions, such as regulating fluid and electrolyte balance, managing blood pressure, and excreting waste products.

A major benefit of kidney detoxification is the reduction of kidney stone formation. Kidney stones are formed when substances such as calcium, oxalate, and phosphate accumulate and crystallize in the kidneys, obstructing the urinary tract and causing pain and discomfort. A proper kidney detox helps break down these crystals and prevent the conditions that cause stones to form, such as dehydration and a diet high in salt and processed foods.

Furthermore, regular detoxing can help prevent the accumulation of metabolic waste products in the blood. In the early stages of kidney disease, the kidneys become less efficient at removing waste like urea and creatinine. By supporting kidney health with detoxification practices, individuals can slow the progression of kidney disease and prevent further damage to kidney tissues.

Additionally, detoxifying the kidneys may also have a positive impact on other body systems. It has been linked to improvements in blood circulation, immune function, and even the health of the skin. The kidneys are responsible for removing toxins from the blood, so when they are operating at full capacity, the body's detoxification process is more efficient, benefiting other organs as well.

2.3 COMMON TOXINS THAT STRAIN YOUR KIDNEYS

While the kidneys are highly efficient at filtering toxins, the modern environment is full of substances that can overwhelm their natural detoxification processes. Common toxins that strain the kidneys include both external chemicals and those produced within the body as part of normal metabolism.

1. **Medications and Over-the-Counter Drugs**: Many medications, including nonsteroidal anti-inflammatory drugs (NSAIDs), certain antibiotics, and pain relievers, can put a strain on the kidneys if taken over long periods of time. These drugs can lead to acute kidney injury (AKI) or chronic kidney disease (CKD) if they accumulate in the bloodstream and are not properly filtered. Additionally, long-term use of certain medications can damage the nephrons and impair the kidneys' filtration abilities.

2. **Heavy Metals**: Exposure to heavy metals such as lead, mercury, and cadmium can be toxic to the kidneys. These metals can accumulate in the body over time and lead to kidney damage. Heavy metal poisoning can disrupt kidney function by interfering with the detoxification process, causing oxidative stress, inflammation, and damage to kidney cells.

3. **Environmental Pollutants**: Air pollution, pesticides, and industrial chemicals are other common toxins that can enter the body through inhalation, ingestion, or skin absorption. These substances are filtered by the kidneys, and prolonged exposure to them can contribute

to kidney stress, oxidative damage, and increased risk of kidney disease. Pollutants such as benzene, toluene, and other volatile organic compounds can accumulate in the bloodstream, overwhelming the kidneys' ability to filter them out effectively.

4. **Dietary Toxins**: Diets that are high in salt, refined sugars, artificial additives, and unhealthy fats can put extra pressure on the kidneys. These substances increase blood pressure, promote fluid retention, and elevate the risk of kidney stones. Excessive salt intake, for example, can lead to fluid retention, which makes the kidneys work harder to maintain electrolyte balance. Moreover, excessive sugar and fat intake can lead to diabetes and obesity, which are major risk factors for kidney disease.

5. **Toxins from Cellular Metabolism**: The body naturally produces waste products as part of its metabolic processes, such as urea, creatinine, and uric acid. These substances are byproducts of protein metabolism and muscle breakdown. If the kidneys are not functioning properly, these waste products can accumulate in the bloodstream, causing toxicity and contributing to kidney damage. Elevated levels of these substances in

the blood are often indicators of impaired kidney function.

6. **Dehydration**: While not a toxin in itself, dehydration can lead to the accumulation of waste products in the kidneys. When the body does not have enough water, urine becomes more concentrated, increasing the risk of kidney stones and impairing the kidneys' ability to filter toxins effectively. Chronic dehydration can lead to kidney damage over time, increasing the risk of CKD.

CHAPTER THREE

NUTRITION FOR KIDNEY REPAIR AND
MAINTENANCE

3.1 THE BEST FOODS FOR KIDNEY HEALTH

A balanced, nutrient-rich diet is essential for kidney repair and maintenance. Certain foods can actively support kidney function by reducing the burden on these vital organs, providing essential vitamins and minerals, and promoting overall health. While individual nutritional needs may vary depending on kidney health and disease progression, some general foods are especially beneficial for kidney repair.

- **Fruits and Vegetables**: Fresh fruits and vegetables are high in fiber, vitamins, minerals, and antioxidants, which support kidney health by reducing inflammation and oxidative stress. Vegetables such as kale, spinach, and bell peppers are packed with antioxidants and essential nutrients like vitamins A, C, and K, which help to protect the kidneys from oxidative damage. Low-potassium fruits like apples, berries, and pears are excellent choices, as they provide vitamins and fiber while maintaining potassium levels within a safe range for individuals with kidney disease.

- **Berries**: Blueberries, strawberries, and raspberries are particularly beneficial for kidney health because they are rich in antioxidants, which help fight free radicals that contribute to kidney damage. Berries also contain vitamin C, fiber, and flavonoids that support the kidneys' detoxification functions. Their anti-inflammatory properties can assist in reducing the risk of kidney inflammation, which can lead to damage over time.

- **Leafy Greens**: Vegetables like kale, spinach, and collard greens are packed with vitamins A, C, and K, and are high in fiber. They are also an excellent source of magnesium, which helps regulate blood pressure, a key factor in preventing kidney disease. However, individuals with advanced kidney disease should monitor potassium intake, as some leafy greens are high in this mineral.

- **Whole Grains**: Whole grains like quinoa, brown rice, and oats are rich in fiber, B vitamins, and antioxidants. These grains help maintain healthy blood sugar levels and reduce the risk of chronic kidney disease (CKD). Fiber is particularly important because it helps regulate blood sugar levels, reducing the strain on the kidneys and preventing kidney damage associated with diabetes.

- **Omega-3 Fatty Acids**: Omega-3 fatty acids, found in foods such as fatty fish (salmon, mackerel, sardines), flaxseeds, and walnuts, have anti-inflammatory effects that can benefit kidney function. They help reduce inflammation in the kidneys and may help prevent the progression of kidney disease. Omega-3s also improve cardiovascular health by lowering blood pressure and cholesterol levels, both of which are vital for kidney health.

- **Garlic and Onion**: Garlic and onions contain sulfur compounds that promote the detoxification processes in the body. These compounds have been shown to reduce inflammation and protect the kidneys from damage. Garlic, in particular, is also known for its ability to lower blood pressure, which can reduce the risk of kidney damage in individuals with hypertension.

- **Olive Oil**: Olive oil is a healthy fat choice that provides antioxidants and polyphenols that help protect the kidneys from oxidative stress and inflammation. It is an excellent alternative to unhealthy fats found in processed and fried foods. Olive oil is also heart-healthy, reducing the risk of heart disease, which often accompanies kidney disease.

- **Low-fat Dairy**: For those who tolerate dairy, low-fat or fat-free options like yogurt and milk can be beneficial for kidney health. Dairy products provide calcium and vitamin D, which help maintain bone health. This is particularly important in kidney disease, as the kidneys play a key role in calcium metabolism.

3.2   HYDRATION: THE KEY TO KIDNEY FUNCTION

Proper hydration is crucial for kidney health, as the kidneys depend on water to perform their filtration and detoxification functions. Water helps to flush out toxins, waste products, and excess substances from the body through urine, ensuring that the kidneys are not overburdened. Hydration also helps prevent kidney stones, urinary tract infections (UTIs), and other kidney-related conditions.

- **How Hydration Affects Kidney Function**: When the body is adequately hydrated, the kidneys can efficiently filter waste and regulate fluid and electrolyte balance. Proper hydration allows for the smooth flow of urine, which helps prevent the build-up of substances like calcium, oxalate, and uric acid—compounds that can form kidney stones when concentrated. Staying hydrated also reduces the risk of kidney infections by flushing out bacteria before it can cause harm.

- **Dehydration and Kidney Health**: On the other hand, dehydration can have a detrimental effect on kidney function. When there is not enough water in the body, the kidneys struggle to remove waste, leading to an accumulation of toxins in the bloodstream. Chronic dehydration can lead to kidney damage, increasing the risk of kidney stones, kidney infections, and even chronic kidney disease. Additionally, dehydration can result in the thickening of urine, which further increases the risk of stone formation and the strain placed on the kidneys.

- **How Much Water Do You Need?**: The amount of water an individual needs depends on several factors, including age, activity level, climate, and kidney health. In general, a good rule of thumb is to aim for about 8 glasses (2 liters) of water a day, though individuals with kidney disease may need more specific recommendations from their healthcare provider. People with advanced kidney disease might need to adjust their fluid intake to avoid excessive fluid buildup, but for most individuals, maintaining adequate hydration is essential.

- **Hydrating Foods**: In addition to drinking water, certain foods can contribute to hydration. Cucumbers, watermelon, strawberries, and celery are all high-water-content foods that can help keep the body hydrated. These foods also provide essential vitamins, minerals, and antioxidants that support kidney function.

3.3 AVOIDING KIDNEY-DAMAGING FOODS AND HABITS

While eating foods that promote kidney health is important, it's equally crucial to avoid foods and habits that can damage the kidneys over time. Certain foods and lifestyle choices can put a strain on the kidneys, especially for individuals with pre-existing kidney disease or those at risk.

- **Excessive Sodium (Salt)**: High salt intake is one of the most damaging factors for kidney health. Excessive sodium can lead to high blood pressure, which is a leading cause of kidney disease. When the kidneys are constantly exposed to high levels of sodium, they become less efficient at regulating fluid balance and waste elimination. Reducing sodium intake by avoiding processed foods, fast food, canned soups, and salty snacks is vital for protecting kidney function.

- **High-Protein Diets**: While protein is essential for the body, excessive protein intake can be hard on the kidneys, particularly for individuals with kidney disease. The breakdown of protein creates waste products that the kidneys must filter out. Consuming large amounts of protein from animal sources (meat, dairy) can increase the kidneys' workload, leading to kidney damage over time. Opting for plant-based protein sources, such as beans, lentils, and tofu, can provide the necessary nutrients without overburdening the kidneys.

- **Refined Sugars and Processed Foods**: Diets high in refined sugars and processed foods are detrimental to kidney health. These foods can contribute to obesity, diabetes, and high blood pressure, all of which are risk factors for kidney disease. Excess sugar can also lead to high blood sugar levels, which put additional strain on the kidneys over time. Reducing the consumption of sugary drinks, sweets, and processed snacks can help protect kidney function.

- **Trans Fats and Unhealthy Oils**: Trans fats and unhealthy oils found in fried foods, baked goods, and margarine can increase the risk of kidney disease by contributing to heart disease, high cholesterol, and inflammation. The kidneys are highly sensitive to inflammation, and consuming inflammatory foods can exacerbate kidney damage. Instead, choose healthy fats, such as those from olive oil, avocado, and nuts, which are easier on the kidneys and promote heart health.

- **Excessive Alcohol**: While moderate alcohol consumption may not pose a significant threat to kidney health in healthy individuals, excessive alcohol intake can lead to kidney damage over time. Alcohol can cause dehydration, increase blood pressure, and interfere with kidney function, particularly in individuals with pre-existing kidney disease. Limiting alcohol consumption is important for preserving kidney health.

- **Smoking**: Smoking is another harmful habit that can have a significant negative impact on kidney health. It contributes to high blood pressure, poor circulation, and reduced oxygen supply to the kidneys, all of which can accelerate the progression of kidney disease. Quitting smoking is one of the most effective ways to protect kidney function and improve overall health.

CHAPTER FOUR

HERBS AND NATURAL SUPPLEMENTS FOR KIDNEY SUPPORT

4.1 BENEFICIAL HERBS FOR KIDNEY HEALTH

Herbs have been used for centuries to support kidney health, prevent kidney disease, and aid in detoxification. Many herbs contain compounds with antioxidant, anti-inflammatory, and diuretic properties, which can be beneficial for the kidneys. Here are some of the most well-known and widely used herbs for kidney health:

- **Dandelion (Taraxacum officinale)**: Dandelion is one of the most commonly used herbs for kidney health. It is a natural diuretic, helping to increase urine production and flush toxins out of the body. Dandelion also contains high levels of potassium, which is important for maintaining fluid balance and supporting kidney function. The herb is rich in antioxidants, which help reduce oxidative stress in the kidneys. Dandelion can be consumed as a tea, supplement, or added to salads and other dishes.

- **Nettle (Urtica dioica)**: Nettle is another powerful herb for kidney health. It has natural diuretic properties, helping to reduce fluid retention and support the kidneys in flushing out waste products. Nettle is also rich in vitamins, minerals, and antioxidants, which support kidney function and reduce inflammation. Studies have shown that nettle can help alleviate symptoms of benign prostatic hyperplasia (BPH) in men, and may have protective effects on the kidneys in conditions like chronic kidney disease (CKD).

- **Horsetail (Equisetum arvense)**: Horsetail is known for its high silica content, which supports connective tissue health, including that of the kidneys. It is also a natural diuretic, promoting increased urine production and aiding in the removal of excess fluid from the body. The herb's diuretic effects can help reduce kidney stone formation by preventing the buildup of minerals in the kidneys. Horsetail is available in herbal tea form, supplements, or tinctures.

- **Ginger (Zingiber officinale)**: Ginger is a well-known anti-inflammatory herb that can help reduce kidney inflammation caused by oxidative stress or kidney disease. It also has diuretic properties and can support kidney detoxification by promoting increased urine production. Ginger is often used in traditional medicine to improve circulation and reduce symptoms of nausea and pain. Fresh ginger can be added to meals, consumed as tea, or taken as a supplement.

- **Cranberry (Vaccinium macrocarpon)**: Cranberries are not only beneficial for urinary tract health but also play a key role in supporting kidney function. They are rich in antioxidants, particularly proanthocyanidins, which help prevent bacteria from sticking to the walls of the urinary tract and kidneys, reducing the risk of infections and promoting kidney health. Cranberries also help to balance urinary pH and prevent kidney stone formation. They can be consumed as fresh berries, juice, or supplements.

- **Turmeric (Curcuma longa)**: Turmeric contains curcumin, a powerful anti-inflammatory and antioxidant compound that supports kidney health by reducing oxidative stress and inflammation. Curcumin has been shown to have protective effects on the kidneys, particularly in individuals with kidney disease. Turmeric can be added to meals or consumed as a supplement, or taken as a tea in combination with other herbs.

- **Parsley (Petroselinum crispum)**: Parsley is often used as a diuretic and kidney tonic. It helps promote urine production and aids in detoxifying the kidneys. Parsley also has anti-inflammatory properties that can reduce kidney inflammation. It is rich in antioxidants, vitamins, and minerals, including vitamin C, which support kidney health. Fresh parsley can be added to meals, or parsley tea can be made by steeping fresh parsley leaves in hot water.

4.2 NATURAL SUPPLEMENTS THAT AID KIDNEY DETOX

In addition to herbs, several natural supplements can support kidney detoxification and improve overall kidney function. These supplements are rich in vitamins, minerals, and antioxidants that promote kidney health by reducing oxidative stress, inflammation, and supporting the kidneys' filtration abilities.

- **Alpha-Lipoic Acid (ALA)**: Alpha-lipoic acid is a powerful antioxidant that helps protect the kidneys from oxidative damage. It supports kidney detoxification by neutralizing free radicals that can cause harm to kidney tissues. ALA also has anti-inflammatory properties, which can reduce kidney inflammation and help in the prevention of kidney disease. It is often taken as a supplement to improve kidney function, particularly in individuals with diabetes-related kidney damage.

- **Coenzyme Q10 (CoQ10)**: CoQ10 is a compound that plays a crucial role in energy production within cells and is also a potent antioxidant. CoQ10 has been shown to support kidney function by improving the health of kidney cells and reducing oxidative damage. It may also help in lowering blood pressure, which is essential for maintaining kidney health. CoQ10 is available in supplement form and can be taken to promote overall kidney health and repair.

- **Vitamin D**: Vitamin D is essential for kidney health because it helps regulate calcium and phosphate balance in the body. The kidneys are responsible for converting vitamin D into its active form, which supports bone health and helps maintain a healthy immune system. In individuals with kidney disease, vitamin D deficiencies are common, so supplementation may be necessary to ensure adequate levels. Vitamin D supplementation can help reduce the risk of complications such as bone disease and cardiovascular issues.

- **Magnesium**: Magnesium is a vital mineral that helps regulate blood pressure, a key factor in kidney health. It also supports kidney function by promoting the excretion of waste products and supporting the kidneys' detoxification abilities. Magnesium is often used to reduce the risk of kidney stone formation and to support kidney health in people with hypertension. Magnesium supplements are available in various forms, including magnesium citrate, magnesium glycinate, and magnesium oxide.

- **Milk Thistle (Silybum marianum)**: Milk thistle is a potent liver detoxifier, but it also supports kidney health due to its anti-inflammatory and antioxidant properties. It contains silymarin, a compound known for its ability to protect kidney cells from oxidative stress. Milk thistle can be particularly useful for individuals with kidney disease or those at risk of kidney damage due to medications or toxins. It is available in capsules or liquid extracts.

- **L-Carnitine**: L-carnitine is an amino acid that plays a critical role in energy production and detoxification. It supports kidney function by improving mitochondrial function within kidney cells and promoting the elimination of waste products. L-carnitine is often used in kidney dialysis patients to improve overall health and reduce fatigue. It is available in supplement form.

- **Omega-3 Fatty Acids**: Omega-3 fatty acids, found in fish oil, flaxseed, and chia seeds, have anti-inflammatory properties that benefit kidney health. Omega-3s help lower blood pressure, reduce inflammation in the kidneys, and improve kidney function. Omega-3 supplements are commonly used to support kidney health, particularly in individuals with chronic kidney disease or those at risk of kidney dysfunction.

4.3 HOW TO SAFELY USE HERBS AND SUPPLEMENTS

While herbs and supplements can be beneficial for kidney health, it is important to use them safely and effectively.

Here are some key guidelines for using herbs and supplements to support kidney function:

- **Consult with a Healthcare Provider**: Before starting any herbal or supplement regimen, it is essential to consult with a healthcare provider, especially for individuals with pre-existing kidney conditions or those taking medications. Some herbs and supplements can interact with medications, and certain herbs may be contraindicated for people with kidney disease.

- **Start with Low Doses**: When using herbs or supplements for kidney health, it is advisable to start with a low dose and gradually increase it, as recommended by a healthcare provider. This allows the body to adjust and helps prevent any adverse reactions.

- **Choose High-Quality Supplements**: Not all herbal supplements are created equal. It is important to choose high-quality supplements from reputable manufacturers to ensure the products are free from contaminants and are properly dosed. Look for supplements that are standardized to contain the correct amount of active ingredients.

- **Avoid Excessive Dosages**: While herbs and supplements can be beneficial, it is crucial not to overuse them. High doses of certain herbs, like dandelion or nettle, can lead to electrolyte imbalances or other adverse effects. Always follow the recommended dosage instructions on the label, and never exceed the prescribed amount without guidance from a healthcare provider.

- **Monitor Kidney Function**: If you are using herbs or supplements to support kidney health, it is important to monitor kidney function regularly through blood tests. This helps ensure that the kidneys are responding well to the supplementation and that no negative side effects are occurring.

- **Be Aware of Potential Side Effects**: Some herbs and supplements can cause side effects, especially when used improperly or in large quantities. For example, excessive use of diuretics like dandelion or nettle can lead to dehydration and electrolyte imbalances. Always be mindful of how your body reacts to the supplements, and discontinue use if any adverse symptoms arise.

CHAPTER FIVE

DETOXIFICATION PRACTICES AND STRATEGIES

5.1 GENTLE DETOX METHODS FOR KIDNEY HEALTH

Detoxification is an important process for kidney health, as the kidneys play a central role in filtering out toxins from the body. However, detoxification should be done gently and in a way that supports kidney function rather than putting additional strain on these vital organs. Gentle detox methods help remove accumulated toxins without overwhelming the kidneys, allowing them to function more efficiently. Here are several gentle detox techniques to consider:

Hydration: One of the simplest and most effective ways to support kidney detoxification is by ensuring proper hydration. Water is essential for the kidneys to flush out toxins, excess salt, and waste products from the body. Drinking enough water helps maintain the kidneys' filtration system, promoting urine production and preventing dehydration. Aim for at least 8 glasses (2 liters) of water per day, though the exact amount can vary depending on factors like age, climate, and activity level.

Herbal Teas: Drinking herbal teas that support kidney health is another gentle detox method. Herbs like dandelion root, nettle, ginger, and parsley have natural diuretic properties that help promote urine production, flushing out toxins and reducing the burden on the kidneys. These herbs also have anti-inflammatory and antioxidant properties, which help reduce oxidative stress and inflammation in the kidneys. Herbal teas can be consumed throughout the day as a mild, soothing detoxification strategy.

Sauna and Sweating: Sweating is another natural way to detoxify the body, as it helps expel toxins through the skin. Using a sauna or engaging in activities that make you sweat, such as exercise, can support kidney detoxification without placing excessive stress on the kidneys. This method also helps with circulation and lymphatic drainage, which further promotes the removal of toxins. It is important to stay hydrated when sweating to replace the fluids lost through perspiration and prevent dehydration.

Dry Brushing: Dry brushing is a technique that involves using a soft brush to stimulate the skin and improve circulation. This process helps to remove dead skin cells and stimulates the lymphatic system, aiding in the removal of toxins. While not directly affecting the kidneys, dry brushing supports overall detoxification by improving the body's ability to eliminate waste through the skin.

Gentle Exercise: Moderate physical activity can promote detoxification by improving circulation and encouraging the elimination of waste through sweat and urine. Activities like walking, yoga, swimming, and cycling are excellent ways to stimulate lymphatic flow and help the body detoxify naturally. However, it's important to avoid overexertion, especially if you have existing kidney issues, as intense exercise can stress the kidneys.

Mindful Eating: Eating a balanced, whole-food diet is a gentle way to support kidney detoxification. Focusing on nutrient-dense foods such as fruits, vegetables, whole grains, and lean proteins provides the body with the vitamins, minerals, and antioxidants it needs to optimize kidney function. Avoiding processed foods, refined sugars, and excess salt helps reduce the burden on the kidneys, enabling them to work more effectively.

5.2 JUICING, FASTING, AND CLEANSING TECHNIQUES

Juicing, fasting, and cleansing are popular detox practices that can support kidney health when done appropriately. These techniques involve consuming specific foods or drinks that help detoxify the body and remove waste products. However, it is important to approach these practices with care, as excessive fasting or cleansing can sometimes be harsh on the kidneys.

- **Juicing**: Juicing is a method of extracting the nutrients from fruits and vegetables in liquid form, allowing the body to absorb vitamins, minerals, and antioxidants quickly. Juices made from ingredients like celery, cucumber, ginger, lemon, and beets are particularly beneficial for kidney detoxification. Celery and cucumber are hydrating and contain compounds that help reduce inflammation and promote urine production. Beet juice, known for its detoxifying effects on the liver, also supports kidney health by improving circulation and flushing toxins from the body.

Juicing can be used as a way to gently cleanse the kidneys, but it should not replace whole meals for long periods of time. A balanced approach, incorporating juices into a well-rounded diet, is the best way to promote kidney health without compromising nutrition. Additionally, it's important to use fresh, organic produce and avoid added sugars or artificial ingredients that can negatively impact kidney function.

- **Fasting**: Fasting is the practice of abstaining from food for a period of time to give the digestive system and other organs a chance to rest and detoxify. Intermittent fasting (where food is restricted to certain windows of time) has gained popularity as a way to support detoxification. During fasting, the body shifts from using glucose for energy to burning fat, a process known as ketosis, which can promote cellular repair and detoxification.

However, fasting can be taxing on the kidneys, especially for individuals with pre-existing kidney conditions. For healthy individuals, short-term intermittent fasting (e.g., 12 to 16 hours) can offer detox benefits by reducing inflammation and allowing the body to remove accumulated toxins. If fasting for longer periods, it's important to stay hydrated and to avoid nutrient deficiencies by reintroducing a well-balanced diet afterward. Anyone with kidney disease or other medical conditions should consult with a healthcare provider before beginning a fasting regimen.

- **Cleansing Techniques**: Kidney cleansing is a practice that involves using specific herbs, teas, or juices to help detoxify the kidneys and promote the elimination of waste. A popular kidney cleansing regimen involves drinking a combination of lemon juice, water, and apple cider vinegar, which may help balance the pH of the body and improve kidney function. Other cleanses may include the use of specific herbs or foods, such as cilantro, cranberry, or watermelon, to support kidney health and promote the removal of toxins.

While kidney cleansing can be beneficial in promoting detoxification, it is essential to ensure that the cleanse does not place undue stress on the kidneys. Many cleansing protocols can be extreme and involve prolonged periods of fasting or consuming only certain foods or liquids. A gentle, short-term cleanse (lasting a few days to a week) can be helpful, but it's important to approach these methods with caution, especially for individuals with kidney disease or other chronic health conditions.

5.3 WHEN TO DETOX AND HOW TO AVOID OVERDOING IT

While detoxification can support kidney health, it's important to recognize when detox practices are appropriate and how to avoid overdoing it. The body has natural detoxification mechanisms, and the kidneys are incredibly efficient at eliminating waste when supported by proper nutrition, hydration, and lifestyle practices. Detoxification should not be seen as a panacea, but rather as a complementary approach to maintaining overall health.

- **Signs You May Need to Detox**: Detoxification may be beneficial when you experience symptoms of toxin buildup in the body, such as fatigue, skin problems, digestive issues, headaches, or general malaise. If you have been exposed to environmental toxins, have a history of poor dietary habits, or are feeling sluggish and unwell, a gentle detox could be helpful. However, if you have chronic kidney disease, or any other serious medical condition, you should consult with a healthcare provider before attempting any detoxification regimen.

- **Avoiding Overdoing It**: Detoxification can be beneficial, but it's important not to overwhelm the body with extreme measures. Overdoing detox practices, such as prolonged fasting, excessive juicing, or harsh cleansing, can strain the kidneys and other organs. The key to a successful detox is balance. Gentle, sustainable methods such as staying hydrated, eating a nutrient-rich diet, and incorporating light detox practices like herbal teas or moderate exercise are usually sufficient for supporting kidney function without causing harm.

- **Resting the Body**: Detoxification should not be a continuous process. The body needs time to rest and recover from detox practices. Frequent, intense detox regimens can lead to nutrient imbalances, dehydration, or fatigue, all of which can put strain on the kidneys and other organs. It's best to limit detox activities to short periods (e.g., a few days or a week) and give your body ample time to rest in between.

- **Consulting a Healthcare Provider**: Before beginning any detox plan, particularly if you have a pre-existing medical condition, it's crucial to consult with a healthcare provider. This is especially important if you are taking medications or have kidney disease, as certain detox practices could interfere with your treatment or worsen your condition. A healthcare provider can help guide you in choosing safe and appropriate detox methods.

CHAPTER SIX

LIFESTYLE FACTORS THAT INFLUENCE KIDNEY HEALTH

6.1 THE IMPACT OF EXERCISE ON KIDNEY FUNCTION

Regular physical activity has a profound effect on overall health, including kidney function. The kidneys play a critical role in filtering waste, regulating fluid balance, and controlling blood pressure. Maintaining optimal kidney health is essential, and exercise is one of the most effective ways to support these processes. Physical activity benefits kidney health in several ways, from improving circulation to managing blood pressure and reducing the risk of chronic kidney disease (CKD).

Improved Circulation and Blood Flow: One of the primary ways exercise supports kidney function is by improving circulation. When we engage in physical activity, the heart pumps blood more efficiently throughout the body, including the kidneys. Enhanced circulation helps the kidneys receive adequate oxygen and nutrients to perform their vital filtration tasks. This increased blood flow can help the kidneys clear waste products more effectively, reducing the burden on these organs.

Blood Pressure Management: Regular exercise is one of the most effective ways to control high blood pressure, a leading cause of kidney damage and a major risk factor for CKD. Physical activity helps lower blood pressure by improving heart health, increasing vascular flexibility, and reducing arterial stiffness. By maintaining a healthy blood pressure range, exercise reduces the strain on the kidneys, lowering the risk of hypertension-related kidney disease. Aerobic exercises like walking, jogging, swimming, and cycling are particularly beneficial for blood pressure regulation.

Managing Diabetes: Type 2 diabetes is another major risk factor for kidney disease. Consistent physical activity helps regulate blood sugar levels by improving insulin sensitivity and encouraging the use of glucose for energy. By reducing insulin resistance, exercise can help prevent or delay the onset of diabetic kidney disease. Activities such as strength training and aerobic exercises are particularly effective in stabilizing blood sugar levels.

Reducing Inflammation and Oxidative Stress: Chronic inflammation and oxidative stress are common contributors to kidney damage. Exercise has been shown to have anti-inflammatory effects, which can reduce the long-term risk of kidney disease. Regular physical activity also helps combat oxidative stress by increasing the body's production of antioxidants, which help neutralize harmful free radicals in the bloodstream. This can reduce the damage done to kidney tissues and improve overall kidney function.

Maintaining a Healthy Weight: Obesity is a significant risk factor for CKD, and maintaining a healthy weight through exercise is one of the best ways to reduce this risk. Being overweight or obese can lead to increased levels of inflammation, high blood pressure, and diabetes, all of which can contribute to kidney damage. Regular exercise, combined with a balanced diet, helps maintain a healthy weight and lowers the risk of kidney disease.

While exercise is essential for kidney health, it's important to avoid overexertion, especially for those with existing kidney conditions. Intense, prolonged exercise without proper hydration can put stress on the kidneys, leading to dehydration and potential kidney damage. It's essential to listen to your body and consult with a healthcare provider before beginning any new exercise program, particularly if you have any pre-existing kidney issues.

6.2 REDUCING STRESS AND ITS EFFECT ON KIDNEYS

Stress is a normal part of life, but chronic stress can have significant adverse effects on overall health, including kidney function. The kidneys are closely connected to the body's stress response system, and prolonged or intense stress can negatively affect kidney health in various ways.

Stress and the Renin-Angiotensin-Aldosterone System (RAAS): The body's stress response involves the activation of the renin-angiotensin-aldosterone system (RAAS), which regulates blood pressure, fluid balance, and electrolyte levels. When the body is under stress, the RAAS system is activated, leading to an increase in blood pressure and fluid retention. While this is helpful in acute stress situations (such as during a fight-or-flight response), chronic activation of this system can lead to sustained high blood pressure (hypertension), which is a leading cause of kidney damage and kidney disease.

Increased Inflammation and Oxidative Stress: Chronic stress can lead to the release of stress hormones such as cortisol, which, over time, can increase inflammation in the body. Inflammation can damage kidney tissues and accelerate the progression of kidney disease. Additionally, stress can contribute to oxidative stress, which harms the kidneys by increasing the number of free radicals in the bloodstream. This can cause long-term kidney damage if stress is not managed effectively.

Stress-Induced Lifestyle Habits: When under stress, people often adopt unhealthy lifestyle habits such as poor eating habits, lack of physical activity, excessive alcohol consumption, and smoking—all of which negatively impact kidney function. Stress can also contribute to poor sleep patterns, which further exacerbate the negative effects on kidney health. Managing stress through healthy coping mechanisms is crucial to prevent these secondary effects on the kidneys.

The Importance of Stress Management: Managing stress is crucial for maintaining kidney health and overall well-being. Various stress-reduction techniques can be effective in lowering stress levels and improving kidney function:

- **Mindfulness and Meditation**: Practicing mindfulness and meditation can help activate the parasympathetic nervous system, which counteracts the body's stress response. Regular meditation has been shown to reduce cortisol levels, lower blood pressure, and improve overall health.

- **Breathing Exercises**: Deep breathing exercises, such as diaphragmatic breathing, can help calm the nervous system and lower stress levels. Focusing on slow, deep breaths can trigger the body's relaxation response and lower cortisol production.

- **Yoga and Tai Chi**: Both yoga and Tai Chi combine mindful movement, deep breathing, and relaxation, helping to reduce stress while improving physical and mental health. These practices can promote kidney health by enhancing circulation, reducing inflammation, and improving overall well-being.

- **Regular Physical Activity**: Exercise, as previously mentioned, is an excellent way to reduce stress. It triggers the release of endorphins, the body's natural "feel-good" hormones, which help alleviate stress and improve mood.

- **Adequate Rest and Sleep**: Ensuring adequate sleep and rest is also a key factor in managing stress. The body needs sufficient sleep to recover from daily stressors and support immune function, hormone regulation, and kidney health.

By managing stress effectively, individuals can prevent the negative impacts of chronic stress on kidney function and improve overall health.

6.3 SLEEP, REST, AND KIDNEY RECOVERY

Sleep and rest are vital for overall health and play an important role in supporting kidney recovery and maintaining kidney function. The body's repair processes, including kidney recovery, occur primarily during restful sleep, making quality sleep essential for those looking to maintain or improve kidney health.

The Role of Sleep in Kidney Health: During sleep, the body undergoes various restorative processes, including cellular repair and waste removal. The kidneys, like other organs, need time to recover from the daily wear and tear that occurs from filtering blood and eliminating waste. Poor sleep or insufficient rest can impair these processes and potentially lead to kidney damage over time.

Sleep and Blood Pressure Regulation: Good quality sleep helps regulate blood pressure, which is essential for kidney health. Hypertension is a major contributor to kidney disease, and sleep deprivation can lead to an increase in blood pressure. Studies have shown that people with sleep apnea or other sleep disorders are at a higher risk of developing high blood pressure, which in turn increases the risk of kidney disease. Ensuring proper sleep can help maintain healthy blood pressure levels and reduce the risk of kidney damage.

The Impact of Sleep on Inflammation: Chronic sleep deprivation has been linked to increased inflammation in the body. Inflammation is a key driver of kidney damage, and sleep plays a crucial role in regulating the body's inflammatory response. Studies have shown that people who sleep less than six hours a night have higher levels of inflammatory markers, which can contribute to the development and progression of kidney disease. Prioritizing sleep helps keep inflammation in check, reducing the burden on the kidneys.

Sleep and Fluid Balance: The kidneys regulate fluid balance in the body, and this process is supported by quality sleep. During sleep, the kidneys work to balance electrolytes and remove waste from the blood. Poor sleep can disrupt the body's natural fluid balance, leading to issues such as fluid retention, dehydration, and impaired kidney function. Ensuring adequate sleep helps the kidneys maintain optimal fluid balance and perform their filtering tasks effectively.

Improving Sleep Quality: To optimize kidney recovery and function, it's important to prioritize good sleep hygiene. Here are some tips for improving sleep quality:

- **Maintain a Consistent Sleep Schedule**: Going to bed and waking up at the same time every day helps regulate the body's internal clock and improves the quality of sleep.
- **Create a Restful Environment**: Make your bedroom a relaxing, sleep-friendly environment by keeping it cool, dark, and quiet. Avoid screens and bright lights at least an hour before bed.
- **Manage Stress**: Practice relaxation techniques before bed to calm the mind and prepare the body for sleep. Meditation, deep breathing exercises, and gentle

stretching can help reduce stress and promote restful sleep.

- **Limit Stimulants**: Avoid consuming caffeine, alcohol, and nicotine close to bedtime, as these substances can interfere with sleep quality and disrupt the body's natural rest cycles.

CHAPTER SEVEN

UNDERSTANDING AND PREVENTING KIDNEY DISEASE

7.1 EARLY SIGNS OF KIDNEY DYSFUNCTION

Kidney disease is often referred to as a "silent" condition because early stages may present few noticeable symptoms. The kidneys are incredibly efficient organs that compensate for their decreased function over time, meaning that kidney dysfunction can progress without overt signs until it becomes more severe. Recognizing early warning signs of kidney problems is crucial for preventing further damage and initiating early treatment. Early intervention can help manage the disease, slow progression, and maintain kidney function for longer.

Changes in Urination: One of the first signs of kidney dysfunction is a change in urination patterns. This could include urinating more frequently, particularly at night (a condition known as nocturia), or experiencing a decrease in urine output. Conversely, some individuals may experience difficulty urinating, or feel the need to urinate urgently without being able to do so. Urine may also appear darker or have a foamy texture, indicating the presence of protein, which is a common sign of kidney damage. If you notice any changes in urination, it is important to consult with a healthcare provider as it may be an early sign of kidney dysfunction.

Swelling in the Extremities: The kidneys are responsible for maintaining a balance of fluids in the body. When kidney function declines, the body may retain excess fluid, leading to swelling (edema) in the ankles, feet, or hands. This is often more noticeable at the end of the day when gravity has caused fluid to accumulate in the lower extremities. Swelling around the eyes, particularly in the morning, is another indicator of kidney problems. If swelling persists or worsens, it's important to seek medical attention.

Fatigue and Weakness: Chronic kidney disease can result in anemia, a condition where the body does not produce enough red blood cells. Red blood cells are necessary for carrying oxygen throughout the body, so when kidney function declines, the body can become deprived of oxygen, leading to fatigue, weakness, and reduced stamina. If you are feeling unusually tired despite getting enough rest, this could be an indication of kidney problems. Additionally, persistent tiredness can interfere with daily activities, and individuals may find themselves feeling constantly drained.

Shortness of Breath: If kidney function deteriorates, the accumulation of fluid in the lungs can lead to shortness of breath, especially when lying down. Difficulty breathing or a sensation of tightness in the chest could indicate fluid overload caused by kidney dysfunction. Anemia associated with kidney disease can also cause shortness of breath, as the body struggles to get enough oxygen to the tissues. If this symptom occurs along with other signs of kidney dysfunction, it is essential to seek medical evaluation.

Back Pain: The kidneys are located at the lower back, just under the rib cage. While back pain is commonly associated with muscle strain or injury, persistent or unexplained pain in this area could be a sign of kidney problems. However, kidney pain is typically dull and deep, rather than sharp or localized like muscle pain. Pain in the back, along with changes in urination or swelling, should be investigated further.

Nausea, Vomiting, and Loss of Appetite: As kidney function declines, waste products build up in the body, causing a condition known as uremia. Uremia can lead to nausea, vomiting, and a general loss of appetite. Individuals with kidney dysfunction may experience a metallic taste in the mouth, making food unappealing. These gastrointestinal symptoms are often overlooked but are a significant sign that the kidneys may not be functioning properly.

High Blood Pressure: The kidneys help regulate blood pressure by controlling fluid balance and producing hormones that help manage the constriction and relaxation of blood vessels. When kidney function is impaired, it can lead to an increase in blood pressure, which can further damage the kidneys in a vicious cycle. High blood pressure is a well-established risk factor for kidney disease, and monitoring blood pressure regularly is crucial, especially for individuals at risk.

7.2 PREVENTIVE MEASURES FOR KIDNEY DISEASE

Preventing kidney disease involves addressing risk factors, adopting healthy lifestyle habits, and ensuring regular monitoring of kidney function. Although kidney disease can sometimes develop despite preventive efforts, taking proactive steps can significantly reduce the risk of developing kidney problems.

Maintaining a Healthy Diet: One of the most effective ways to prevent kidney disease is to maintain a diet that supports kidney health. A balanced diet that is rich in fruits, vegetables, whole grains, and lean proteins helps to reduce the risk of conditions such as high blood pressure, diabetes, and obesity, which are key risk factors for kidney disease. Limiting the intake of salt, processed foods, and high-fat foods can help reduce the strain on the kidneys and prevent fluid retention.

For kidney health, focusing on foods that provide essential nutrients without overloading the kidneys with toxins or excess sodium is important. Foods rich in antioxidants, such as berries, leafy greens, and cruciferous vegetables, can help combat inflammation and oxidative stress, which are implicated in kidney damage.

Regular Exercise: Physical activity is vital for maintaining healthy kidneys. Regular exercise can help manage blood pressure, reduce the risk of diabetes, and improve overall cardiovascular health—all of which are essential for kidney function. The American Kidney Fund recommends at least 150 minutes of moderate-intensity exercise per week, such as walking, swimming, or cycling. Exercise also helps with weight management, reducing the risk of obesity, which is closely linked to kidney disease.

Staying Hydrated: Proper hydration is essential for kidney health, as the kidneys rely on water to filter waste and maintain fluid balance. However, it's important to strike a balance. Drinking too much water can put unnecessary stress on the kidneys, while dehydration can lead to kidney stones or even kidney failure in severe cases. It is generally recommended to drink at least 8 cups (2 liters) of water per day, but individual needs may vary based on activity level, climate, and other factors.

Avoiding Excessive Use of Painkillers: Over-the-counter pain medications such as nonsteroidal anti-inflammatory drugs (NSAIDs), including ibuprofen and naproxen, can damage the kidneys if used excessively or over a prolonged period. It is important to limit the use of these medications and consult a healthcare provider before taking them regularly, especially for individuals with pre-existing kidney conditions.

Monitoring Kidney Function: Regular check-ups with a healthcare provider can help detect early signs of kidney dysfunction. People at higher risk of kidney disease, such as those with a family history of kidney problems, diabetes, high blood pressure, or heart disease, should undergo routine kidney function tests. The most common tests include blood tests to measure creatinine and glomerular filtration rate (GFR), and urine tests to detect protein or blood in the urine, both of which are early indicators of kidney damage.

Avoiding Smoking and Excessive Alcohol Consumption: Smoking and excessive alcohol consumption can increase the risk of kidney disease. Smoking can damage blood vessels, which impairs circulation to the kidneys, while excessive alcohol can lead to dehydration, liver damage, and increased blood pressure. Quitting smoking and limiting alcohol intake can greatly reduce the risk of kidney dysfunction.

Managing Chronic Conditions: Proper management of chronic conditions like diabetes and high blood pressure is essential for preventing kidney disease. People with diabetes should aim to keep blood sugar levels within the recommended range to prevent damage to the kidneys. Similarly, individuals with high blood pressure should take steps to manage their condition, either through lifestyle changes (e.g., diet, exercise) or medications as prescribed by a healthcare provider.

7.3 MANAGING RISK FACTORS AND CHRONIC CONDITIONS

Managing risk factors and chronic conditions is crucial for preventing kidney disease or slowing its progression. Key conditions such as high blood pressure, diabetes, and heart disease can contribute to kidney damage if left untreated. Here's how to effectively manage these conditions:

Managing High Blood Pressure: High blood pressure is one of the leading causes of kidney disease. If left uncontrolled, high blood pressure can damage the blood vessels in the kidneys, making it harder for them to filter waste. To manage blood pressure, individuals should aim for a target of 120/80 mmHg or lower, as recommended by healthcare providers. This can be achieved through lifestyle changes, such as reducing salt intake, exercising regularly, and maintaining a healthy weight. For those with more severe hypertension, medication may be necessary to keep blood pressure under control.

Controlling Blood Sugar Levels: Diabetes is another major risk factor for kidney disease, as it can damage the blood vessels in the kidneys over time. People with diabetes should monitor their blood sugar levels regularly and aim to keep them within the target range. This can be achieved through a combination of diet, exercise, and medication. Additionally, individuals with diabetes should have their kidney function tested regularly to detect any early signs of kidney damage.

Cholesterol Management: High cholesterol can contribute to the development of atherosclerosis (narrowing of the arteries), which can reduce blood flow to the kidneys. Managing cholesterol levels through diet, exercise, and medications (such as statins) can help protect the kidneys from damage.

Avoiding Smoking: Smoking accelerates the progression of kidney disease by narrowing the blood vessels, which reduces blood flow to the kidneys. Quitting smoking is one of the best ways to reduce the risk of kidney damage and slow the progression of existing kidney disease.

Regular Health Screenings: Regular screenings for kidney function, blood pressure, blood sugar levels, and cholesterol are vital for individuals at risk of kidney disease. Early detection allows for prompt intervention, which can prevent or slow the progression of kidney dysfunction.

CHAPTER EIGHT

CONCLUSION: ACHIEVING LONG-TERM KIDNEY HEALTH

8.1 THE ROAD TO KIDNEY RECOVERY AND OPTIMAL FUNCTION

Achieving long-term kidney health requires a comprehensive approach that incorporates proper care, lifestyle changes, and consistent monitoring. The road to kidney recovery and maintaining optimal function is not always straightforward, but with commitment and the right strategies, it is entirely achievable. Whether you are recovering from kidney disease, managing a chronic condition, or aiming to prevent kidney issues, the key is to understand your body's needs and address them proactively.

Early Intervention is Key: The earlier kidney dysfunction is detected, the better the chance for recovery and preservation of kidney function. Regular check-ups, including blood and urine tests to monitor kidney function, are essential for early diagnosis. When kidney problems are detected early, medical treatments combined with lifestyle changes can slow or even reverse some damage. For example, managing high blood pressure or diabetes can prevent further damage to the kidneys, while adopting a kidney-friendly diet can improve kidney function.

Consistent Hydration and Proper Nutrition: Hydration plays a significant role in kidney recovery and optimal function. The kidneys rely on a sufficient amount of water to effectively filter waste from the bloodstream. Ensuring consistent hydration and adopting a balanced diet with nutrient-dense foods that support kidney health is fundamental. Foods high in antioxidants, such as berries and leafy greens, and those low in sodium, can reduce inflammation and prevent the buildup of harmful substances in the body. By making these dietary changes, individuals can support kidney function and enhance their ability to filter waste efficiently.

Medication and Medical Support: For those recovering from kidney disease or managing chronic kidney conditions, medication may be necessary to control symptoms, manage underlying causes, or prevent further damage. Medications such as blood pressure-lowering drugs, diabetes management medications, and diuretics (to reduce fluid retention) are essential in supporting kidney recovery. Working closely with a healthcare provider ensures the appropriate use of these medications and helps monitor kidney function during treatment.

Exercise and Physical Activity: Exercise is also crucial for kidney recovery and optimal function. Regular physical activity improves circulation, helps control blood pressure, and enhances overall well-being. For individuals with chronic kidney disease (CKD), engaging in moderate exercise under medical supervision can increase energy levels, reduce swelling, and improve kidney function. Exercise can also combat obesity, a risk factor for kidney disease, by promoting weight loss and improving metabolic health.

Addressing Underlying Conditions: Many kidney issues arise from underlying conditions like high blood pressure, diabetes, or heart disease. Effectively managing these conditions is essential for the road to kidney recovery. This may involve taking medications, adhering to lifestyle changes, or undergoing regular check-ups. For instance, keeping blood pressure in the normal range and managing blood sugar levels can reduce the strain on the kidneys and protect them from further damage. In some cases, more intensive treatments, such as dialysis, may be required if the kidney disease is advanced. However, even in these cases, lifestyle changes can significantly improve overall quality of life and support kidney health.

8.2 CREATING A SUSTAINABLE KIDNEY HEALTH PLAN

A sustainable kidney health plan is essential for ensuring that kidney function is supported over the long term. A personalized, proactive plan should take into account individual health conditions, risk factors, and goals. Creating such a plan involves setting realistic health goals and adopting habits that promote kidney health while addressing areas of concern.

Comprehensive Lifestyle Changes: The foundation of a sustainable kidney health plan is lifestyle changes. These include regular physical activity, a balanced diet, stress management, adequate hydration, and avoiding harmful habits such as smoking and excessive alcohol consumption. Lifestyle changes should be tailored to individual needs, as no one-size-fits-all approach exists. For example, individuals with diabetes need to monitor their blood sugar levels closely, while those with high blood pressure should focus on reducing sodium intake and engaging in exercises that help lower blood pressure.

Regular Health Monitoring: Kidney health should be monitored consistently through regular check-ups with a healthcare provider. Monitoring kidney function through blood tests, urine analysis, and blood pressure measurements is essential for detecting any early signs of dysfunction. If any abnormalities are found, a plan can be developed to address the issues before they progress to more serious conditions. Regular monitoring allows for early intervention, which is critical for the long-term health of the kidneys.

Managing Chronic Conditions: For those at risk of kidney disease or already dealing with chronic kidney conditions, a sustainable health plan will include a focus on managing underlying conditions like diabetes, hypertension, or heart disease. By consistently managing these conditions through medication, lifestyle changes, and regular monitoring, individuals can protect their kidneys from further damage. For instance, those with diabetes should focus on controlling their blood sugar, while those with hypertension should take steps to keep their blood pressure within healthy limits.

Adopting Kidney-Friendly Diets: A key component of a sustainable kidney health plan is adopting a kidney-friendly diet. This diet typically includes foods rich in antioxidants, healthy fats, and fiber while limiting sodium, processed foods, and excessive protein. For example, focusing on whole, plant-based foods such as vegetables, fruits, nuts, and legumes can reduce inflammation and oxidative stress, two factors that can contribute to kidney damage. It is also crucial to avoid or limit foods that may worsen kidney function, such as processed meats, excess salt, and high-phosphorus foods like soda.

Long-Term Goal Setting: A sustainable kidney health plan should also include long-term goal setting. These goals may involve improving blood pressure, maintaining a healthy weight, reducing the risk of kidney disease, or recovering from kidney injury. Achieving these goals requires consistency and patience, as kidney health is a long-term commitment. Setting small, achievable milestones along the way can help maintain motivation and ensure that progress is being made.

8.3 EMBRACING A HOLISTIC LIFESTYLE FOR LIFELONG WELLNESS

The road to achieving lifelong kidney health is paved with holistic lifestyle choices that extend beyond diet and exercise. A holistic approach involves taking care of the entire body and mind to create a balanced and sustainable life. This approach not only promotes kidney health but also supports overall well-being.

Mind-Body Connection: A holistic approach to kidney health recognizes the important connection between mind and body. Managing stress through mindfulness, meditation, and relaxation techniques can positively influence kidney health. Chronic stress can lead to inflammation, high blood pressure, and poor eating habits, all of which can harm the kidneys. Incorporating practices such as yoga, deep breathing exercises, or meditation can reduce stress levels and improve mental clarity, which, in turn, supports physical health.

Prioritizing Rest and Sleep: Adequate sleep is crucial for kidney health, as it allows the body to rest and repair itself. During sleep, the kidneys work to filter waste, balance fluids, and maintain electrolyte levels. Chronic sleep deprivation can lead to high blood pressure and increased inflammation, both of which are risk factors for kidney disease. Creating a restful sleep environment, following a consistent sleep schedule, and managing stress before bed can improve sleep quality and support kidney recovery.

Environmental Factors: A holistic lifestyle also involves considering environmental factors that may affect kidney health. Reducing exposure to toxins, pollutants, and chemicals is an essential aspect of a kidney health plan. This includes avoiding smoking and limiting exposure to harmful substances such as pesticides, industrial chemicals, and air pollution. Creating a clean and healthy living environment, eating organic foods when possible, and avoiding overuse of harsh chemicals can help protect the kidneys from harmful substances.

Support Systems: Achieving long-term kidney health is easier when individuals have a solid support system. This includes a network of healthcare providers, family, and friends who can offer encouragement and guidance. Having a strong support system can make it easier to stick to a kidney health plan, especially during challenging times. Whether it's participating in group exercise, attending support groups for chronic conditions, or working with a registered dietitian, social support plays a crucial role in maintaining motivation and ensuring success.

Sustaining Lifelong Wellness: Achieving kidney health is not a short-term goal; it is a lifelong journey. By embracing a holistic lifestyle that incorporates healthy eating, regular physical activity, stress management, proper sleep, and environmental awareness, individuals can maintain kidney health throughout their lives. Creating sustainable habits that focus on long-term well-being ensures that kidneys continue to function optimally well into older age, preventing disease and preserving quality of life.

In conclusion, the road to achieving long-term kidney health is built on consistent and mindful efforts. Recovery, prevention, and maintenance of kidney function require a holistic approach that integrates medical care, lifestyle changes, and mental well-being. By creating a sustainable kidney health plan and adopting a balanced lifestyle, individuals can enjoy optimal kidney function and lifelong wellness. With dedication, proactive care, and the right strategies, long-term kidney health is within reach for everyone.